The Sheldon Short Guide to
Liver Disease

Mark Greener spent a decade in biomedical research before joining *MIMS Magazine* for GPs in 1989. Since then, he has written on health and biology for magazines worldwide for patients, healthcare professionals and scientists. He is a member of the Royal Society of Biology and is the author of 21 other books, including *The Heart Attack Survival Guide* (2012) and *The Holistic Health Handbook* (2013), both published by Sheldon Press. Mark lives with his wife, three children and two cats in a Cambridgeshire village.

GW00647811

Sheldon Short Guides

A list of titles in the Overcoming Common Problems series is also available from Sheldon Press, 36 Causton Street, London SW1P 4ST and on our website at www.sheldonpress.co.uk

THE SHELDON
SHORT GUIDE TO
LIVER
DISEASE

Mark Greener

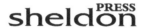

First published in Great Britain in 2016

Sheldon Press
36 Causton Street
London SW1P 4ST
www.sheldonpress.co.uk

British Library Cataloguing-in-Publication Data
A catalogue record for this book is available from the
British Library

ISBN 978-1-84709-386-8
eBook ISBN 978-1-84709-387-5

Typeset by Fakenham Prepress Solutions, Fakenham,
Norfolk NR21 8NN
First printed in Great Britain by Ashford Colour Press
Subsequently digitally reprinted in Great Britain

eBook by Fakenham Prepress Solutions, Fakenham,
Norfolk NR21 8NN

Produced on paper from sustainable forests

616·362

Contents

A note to the reader

This is not a medical book and is not intended to replace advice from your doctor. Consult your pharmacist or doctor if you believe you have any of the symptoms described, and if you think you might need medical help.

A note on references

I used numerous medical and scientific papers to write the book that this Sheldon Short is based on: *Coping with Liver Disease*. Unfortunately, there isn't space to include references in this short summary. You can find these in *Coping with Liver Disease*, which discusses the topics in more detail. I updated some facts and figures for this book.

Introduction

According to Greek legend, Zeus once punished humanity by making us forget how to use fire. Another god, Prometheus, restored this knowledge. In revenge, Zeus chained Prometheus to a rock, while an eagle ate his liver. Prometheus's liver regenerated overnight and the eagle feasted again. Prometheus's torment lasted 13 generations until Heracles slew the eagle.

Remarkably, the legend contains a kernel of truth: the liver's superlative powers of rejuvenation. Indeed, the liver can regain its normal size and function even after a surgeon removes three-quarters of the organ. Yet numerous diseases and unhealthy lifestyles can overwhelm the liver's legendary ability to recover. According to the British Liver Trust (<www.britishlivertrust.org.uk/>), liver disease kills more people than diabetes and road accidents combined.

Typically, liver diseases progress from hepatitis (liver inflammation) to cirrhosis (scarring) to cancer over 20–40 years. So, you can often prevent, or at least delay, serious health problems. This book aims to help you understand liver disease and appreciate the best way to manage symptoms and improve your long-term prospects. I hope that, as well as resolving some immediate issues, this book will inspire further questions, which your doctor, nurse and pharmacist will be happy to answer.

1

Inside a healthy liver

About three weeks after conception, a small bud forms just below the embryo's stomach, which develops into the liver and gall bladder. The liver's size gradually increases. A healthy adult liver typically weighs between 1,200 and 1,500 g.

Normally, a liver has two lobes: the right lobe is about six times larger than the left. Place your right hand over the lower right-hand side of your ribs. Your handprint roughly covers your liver (Figure 1 overleaf). The upper edge of the right lobe is about 1 cm below your right nipple. The upper edge of the liver's left lobe is about 2 cm below your left nipple.

The gall bladder

The pear-shaped gall bladder fills with and concentrates bile, a greenish-yellow fluid produced by the liver. The gall bladder, which lies under the liver and usually stores around 50 ml of bile, contracts when you eat. This pushes bile along tubes called ducts and into the part of your gut called the duodenum, where bile helps you digest fats.

Looking down a microscope at a slice of human liver reveals rows of cells (hepatocytes) radiating from a central vein. Hepatocytes are the liver's main workhorse: a gram of normal liver contains about two million

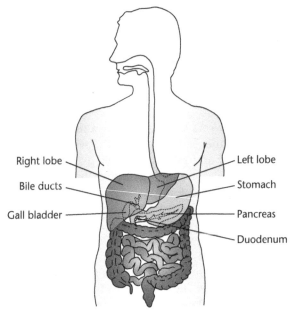

Figure 1 The position of a healthy liver

cells. The liver also contains, for example, Kupffer cells, which remove old and damaged blood cells, debris, bacteria, viruses, parasites and cancer cells. Alcohol damages Kupffer cells.

The body's waste disposal unit

Removing waste is probably the liver's best-known role. Our ancestors (and some people in developing countries even today) often scavenged food from the wild. Sometimes their food was decaying or caked in dirt. Water came from rivers and ponds. So, we evolved formidable defences against the poisons, microbe other chemicals we inevitably consumed.

Ingested food, chemicals and pathogens cross the gut and enter the blood vessels that supply the gastrointestinal tract ('gut'). This blood passes through the liver before reaching the rest of the body. The liver usually breaks down chemicals to less harmful 'metabolites' that the body can remove more easily in bile (and, in turn, faeces) and urine. For example, the liver removes about one unit of alcohol from your blood an hour, although the rate differs dramatically between people. The liver also receives a rich blood supply from the rest of the body. So, the liver can remove harmful by-products of the processes that keep us alive, as well as chemicals that eluded the first filter or that you inhaled.

The liver also filters lymph, a clear, yellowish fluid that bathes your tissues and contains white blood cells, which help you fight infections. That's why your lymph nodes (such as the 'glands' under your chin and in your armpits) may swell when you have an infection.

Supplying our energy demands

Cells are, essentially, biological factories. They use a sugar called glucose as fuel. We extract glucose from carbohydrates (such as sugars and starch) in our diet. But we need to keep our bodies going when food is scarce – or even if it's a while until our next meal.

So, in times of plenty, liver cells stick glucose together into a long chain called glycogen, which stores energy. Glycogen in the liver and muscle stores enough energy to keep an average woman going for about a day. Once glycogen makes up more than about 5 per cent of the liver's weight, production declines.

Our ancestors, however, often did not know where their next meal was coming from. So, liver cells convert the additional glucose into 'fatty acids'. The liver releases fatty acids into the blood when the body needs another source of energy. In times of plenty, fat cells (adipocytes) take up glucose, which they use to make another chemical called glycerol. Adipocytes join glycerol to the fatty acids produced by the liver to form fats called triglycerides. This stores enough energy to keep you going for several weeks. When we've depleted our other energy stores, we start breaking down muscle. This releases the building blocks of protein (amino acids). The liver can convert some amino acids into glucose.

Cholesterol: the misunderstood fat

The liver makes cholesterol, which is part of the membranes surrounding every cell. Cholesterol is also part of the 'myelin sheath' around many nerves that ensures that signals travel properly and forms the backbone of several hormones.

Your body surrounds cholesterol with soluble coats called lipoproteins to aid transport around the body – for instance:

- Low-density lipoprotein (LDL) carries cholesterol from the liver to the tissues. LDL accumulates in artery walls, forming fatty deposits that contribute to heart attacks, some strokes, kidney damage and some other diseases.
- High-density lipoprotein (HDL) carries cholesterol to the liver for removal.

So, high LDL levels increase, and high levels of HDL reduce, the risk of heart attacks and other diseases. It's easy to remember: LDL is 'lethal'; HDL is 'healthy'.

The liver's other actions

The liver has several other critical roles, including:

- making haem: part of haemoglobin, which carries oxygen in red blood cells;
- storing vitamin A, which is important for vision, healthy bones, reproduction and immune responses;
- producing a protein called albumin, which helps balance fluid levels in your body and transports calcium, several hormones and some medicines;
- producing proteins that stop bleeding when we cut ourselves and prevent potentially harmful clots forming inside the body;
- converting the type of vitamin D made by sunlight's action on the skin and from food into the main active circulating form.

This central role in numerous critical biological processes helps explain why liver diseases can prove devastating, debilitating and deadly.

2

Symptoms of liver disease

The liver can compensate for relatively extensive damage. So, symptoms often emerge only once liver disease is already well advanced. Many symptoms of liver disease are, however, easily confused with those of other ailments. Furthermore, the same symptom may arise from different triggers. So, deciding on symptoms alone whether you have liver disease, and if so which

Table 1 Possible symptoms of liver disease

See your GP if you develop any of the following:
    Fatigue and weakness
    Feeling generally unwell
    Loss of appetite
    Nausea, vomiting or both
    Unexplained weight loss (e.g. without dieting)
    Pain or discomfort in the abdomen
    Feeling itchy, especially if severe
    Small red veins that look a bit like a spider (spider naevi)
    Enlarged and tender liver, especially below your right ribs
    Dark, brown urine
    Grey, pale, clay-coloured stools (faeces)
    Loss of sex drive
*See your GP **immediately** if you develop any of the following:*
    Yellow tinge to your skin and eyes (jaundice)
    Swollen abdomen
    Dark or black, tarry faeces
    Fever with high temperature and shivering
    Vomiting blood

Source: Adapted from the British Liver Trust

type and the triggers, is often difficult. But see your GP if you develop any of the symptoms in Table 1.

Cirrhosis

Scars protect an injured area while your body repairs the damage. When damage is short-lived, hepatic scarring helps your liver return to normal. Repeated damage can, however, produce extensive scarring, known as fibrosis. Eventually, hard, irregular areas of scar tissue, called nodules, replace smooth liver. These nodules can hinder blood flow, which can starve liver cells of oxygen and nutrients, resulting in cirrhosis.

Cirrhosis tends to emerge when the liver damage is unrelenting, such as drinking excessively for many years or persistent (chronic) infections with some viruses. For example, up to a quarter of people infected

Table 2 Symptoms of cirrhosis

Tiredness
Weakness
Loss of appetite
Unexplained weight loss
Nausea
Severe itching (pruritus)
Tenderness or pain around your liver
Spider naevi above your waist
Jaundice*
Bleeding problems*
Hair loss
Fever and shivering (the liver damage means you are more likely to pick up a bug)
Oedema (accumulation of fluid in your legs, ankles and feet)
Ascites*

*See the relevant sections elsewhere in this book.

with hepatitis C virus (HCV; page 21) develop cirrhosis. Again, see your GP if you have any symptom in Table 2.

The liver cannot repair cirrhosis. But removing the cause (e.g. stopping drinking or treating HCV) often prevents the cirrhosis from getting worse. In 'compensated' cirrhosis, the liver's spare capacity means that the organ still performs many important tasks. In decompensated cirrhosis, the damage overwhelms the spare capacity, which can cause debilitating symptoms and potentially life-threatening complications. Doctors cannot yet predict accurately who will develop cirrhosis and how the condition will progress. So, you might need regular monitoring.

Itching and liver disease

People with chronic liver disease can suffer severe itching (pruritus). Sometimes pruritis affects one part of the body, such as the hands or feet. Sometimes pruritus is more widespread. The itching seems to arise when the liver cannot remove toxins. Moisturizers, oatmeal baths and some drugs from your doctor may alleviate itching.

Mental changes

People with chronic liver disease can experience mental problems, such as depression and anxiety. Sometimes these arise from the burden imposed by living with liver disease. Sometimes they are a side effect. And, sometimes, they're caused by liver disease. Cirrhosis can, for example, cause 'hepatic encephalopathy' characterized by one or more of:

- personality changes
- altered sleep patterns

- violent behaviour
- sluggish movements
- speech problems
- drowsiness
- confusion and poor mental performance
- stupor
- coma.

Hepatic encephalopathy seems to arise when inflammation spilling out from the liver and high levels of toxins cause certain nerve and other cells in the brain to swell. Meanwhile, the amount of fluid in the brain increases (cerebral oedema).

See your doctor if you experience mental changes. If you have hepatic encephalopathy, your doctor may prescribe a laxative, which may help remove toxins from your body. That's another good reason to eat a high-fibre diet. Hepatic encephalopathy often follows infections, constipation, dehydration, bleeding or treatment with certain medicines. So, your doctor will treat any underlying cause.

Portal hypertension

A blood vessel called the hepatic portal vein carries blood from the gut and spleen to the liver. Your spleen, which is normally about the size of your fist, lies above your stomach and under your ribs on the left side of your body. The spleen, part of your lymphatic system (page 3), has several important roles, including:

- storing white blood cells (which fight infection), red blood cells and platelets (which help blood clot);
- helping to control the amount of blood circulating around your body;
- destroying old and damaged blood cells;

• making red blood cells and some white blood cells (although bone marrow produces most blood cells).

Portal hypertension means that the blood pressure is dangerously high in the hepatic portal vein. Portal hypertension can force blood along smaller vessels to find a way back to the heart, causing them to swell, which potentially forms varices (see page 12). This increased pressure may also mean that the spleen swells with blood. A spleen swollen by portal hypertension is less able to store red and white blood cells. It is also less able to store platelets, which is one reason why people with cirrhosis are particularly likely to experience bleeding problems (page 11).

Other complications of cirrhosis

Cirrhosis can cause other complications, including:

• *Muscle wasting* A cirrhotic liver cannot process proteins effectively.
• *Hormonal changes* The liver regulates levels of some hormones. So, cirrhosis can cause, for example, irregular periods in women and breast enlargement in men. Hormonal changes may weaken the skeleton, contributing to osteoporosis (brittle bone disease), increasing the risk of debilitating fractures.
• *Osteoporosis* As we get older the skeleton's strength naturally declines. Muscle wasting, alcoholism, hormonal changes and low levels of vitamin D hasten the decline. So, consume sufficient vitamin D and calcium. But speak to your doctor first.
• *Kidney disease* Some people with decompensated cirrhosis show poor kidney function, which can contribute to, for example, ascites (see below),

oedema (fluid build-up) in the feet and legs and kidney disorders.

- *Bleeding problems* The liver produces chemicals that help blood clot and the release of platelets from a spleen enlarged by portal hypertension may decline. So, people with cirrhosis may bruise and bleed easily (e.g. suffering frequent nosebleeds or bleeding gums). Your doctor may regularly measure how quickly your blood clots.
- *Jaundice* The spleen destroys old and damaged red blood cells, releasing a yellowish product called bilirubin, which is largely excreted in bile. Faeces' brown colour comes from the conversion of bilirubin into another chemical called stercobilin. You excrete some bilirubin in urine after conversion into urobilin (that's why urine is yellowish). Several liver diseases increase blood levels of bilirubin, potentially triggering jaundice: a yellow tinge to the skin and whites of the eyes. As levels rise, the kidneys excrete more bilirubin and there is less in the faeces. So, urine can turn dark brown. Faeces become pale and clay-coloured.
- *Ascites* Ascites form when fluid builds up between the tissues lining the abdomen and the organs. Cirrhosis squeezes blood vessels inside the liver. So, blood begins to back up and leaks into the abdomen. The accumulation of fluid can leave the person looking heavily pregnant and may press on the diaphragm, causing shortness of breath. Around half of people with cirrhosis develop ascites over a decade. Several cancers can also cause ascites. Doctors may advise that you reduce the amount of salt (which causes water retention) and take diuretics. These make you excrete more urine, reducing

the amount of fluid in your body. In some cases, a surgeon may drain fluid from your abdomen.

- *Varices* Around 60 per cent of people with cirrhosis develop varices, caused when portal hypertension stretches the veins supplying the upper part of the stomach, the lower food pipe and rectum. In severe cases, swollen veins protrude into the oesophagus, forming varices. Some varices slowly leak blood, possibly causing anaemia. Others burst, causing severe bleeding, and you may vomit blood or pass stools streaked with black blood. Between 40 and 45 per cent of those with large varices due to cirrhosis experience at least one bleed a year. Up to half of people who develop bleeding varices die. Go to A&E or call an ambulance if you or someone you know vomits blood. You should see your doctor urgently if you start passing bloody faeces. Apart from liver disease, blood in your stools can be a sign of other diseases, including colon cancer.

Treating varices

Surgeons may treat varices by:

- placing a small band around the varices to stop the bleeding;
- injecting a chemical into the varices to trigger clotting and scarring, which closes the vessel;
- passing a tube with a balloon on the end into the stomach. When inflated, the balloon squeezes the varices, which reduces bleeding;
- joining two larger veins with a metal tube called a stent to bypass the swollen vessel.

Doctors may prescribe drugs to reduce blood pressure (antihypertensives).

End-stage liver disease

Eventually, liver damage can mean that the organ can no longer perform its normal functions (end-stage liver disease), which causes serious symptoms and complications. A liver transplant is often the only effective treatment for end-stage liver disease.

3

Testing for liver disease

Liver diseases often produce rather vague symptoms, which overlap with other conditions. And many people with early liver disease do not develop any symptoms. So, doctors use a variety of tests to help diagnose liver disease.

Virology and immunology

Doctors may take a blood sample to measure molecules produced by the virus or levels of the antibodies made by your body to fight the virus. Measuring levels of the virus (viral load) helps see how well you are responding to treatment. Doctors now regard undetectable levels of HCV (page 21) 12 weeks after the end of antiviral treatment as equivalent to a cure, for example.

Autoimmune diseases

Antibodies help white blood cells recognize and destroy bacteria, viruses, parasites and cancerous cells. However, occasionally antibodies mistakenly attack healthy cells. During primary biliary cirrhosis, for example, this 'autoimmune' attack destroys bile ducts. In autoimmune hepatitis, antibodies attack liver cells. Inflammation caused by other autoimmune diseases – including type 1 diabetes, ulcerative colitis and rheumatoid arthritis – can spill over and inflame the liver. So, doctors may test for autoantibodies.

Imaging

Soft organs, such as the liver, show relatively little detail on X-rays. However, several methods help doctors gain a better view.

- *Angiography* Injecting a 'contrast medium', which absorbs X-rays, outlines blood vessels. So, the X-ray shows changes in blood flow in the liver, which may localize abnormalities, including tumours, and help surgeons plan operations.
- *Ultrasound* machines pick up sound waves as they bounce off tissue and can detect changes in the liver's size and shape as well as revealing fatty deposits (steatosis).
- *Computed tomography (CT)* – sometimes called CAT (computerized axial tomography) scans – uses X-rays to produce numerous 'slices' through your body. A computer rebuilds the slices into a single three-dimensional, high-resolution image. Radiologists may use a contrast medium to enhance fine detail.
- *Magnetic resonance imaging (MRI)* uses powerful magnetic fields to provide an even more detailed view than CT. Both CT and MRI can detect tumours, help detect the cause of jaundice, guide biopsies and so on.

The risks and benefits of liver biopsy

During a biopsy, the doctor takes a small sample of tissue, which is then examined under the microscope or subjected to tests. Biopsies are the most accurate way to diagnose some liver diseases. However, a biopsy can cause bleeding or lead to bile leaking. If you have liver cancer, there is a small risk that the malignancy could spread along the 'tunnel' left by the needle. Discuss the risks and benefits with your doctor.

Laparoscopy

A thin tube with a camera and light at the end is inserted into your abdomen through a small cut to examine your liver. You'll be under a general anaesthetic.

Liver function tests

Liver damage or inflammation can lead to certain enzymes leaking into your bloodstream, which doctors measure during 'liver function tests' (LFTs). Abnormal LFTs do not necessarily indicate liver damage: they can rise after a curry, alcohol or some medicines, for example. Furthermore, not everyone with liver disease shows abnormal LFTs. Your doctor should check whether an abnormal LFT is a 'one-off' or indicates an underlying problem.

4

The A to E of viral hepatitis

Five viruses – hepatitis A to E – can replicate inside, and damage, hepatocytes (page 1). Meanwhile, the immune system targets infected liver cells. This dual attack can cause swelling, inflammation, scarring and, eventually, liver cancer.

Hepatitis A

Hepatitis A virus (HAV) usually spreads from food and drink contaminated with faeces from an infected person when personal hygiene and sanitation are poor. HAV does not cause chronic liver disease and rarely kills. Nevertheless, HAV can cause unpleasant symptoms including:

- fever
- malaise
- poor appetite
- diarrhoea
- nausea
- abdominal discomfort
- jaundice.

Symptoms are more common and more severe in adults than children, but usually subside after a few weeks to several months.

There is no specific treatment. So, prevention is key. If you have HAV, don't share towels and wash your hands thoroughly after going to the toilet and before preparing food, or ask someone else to prepare your family's food. HAV can spread through contact with infected blood: don't share eating utensils, toothbrushes, razors and the equipment ('works') used to inject street drugs. You cannot contract HAV by casual contact.

When travelling to countries with poor sanitation:

- boil drinking water (including water used for brushing teeth) or use bottled water;
- avoid ice, poorly cooked shellfish, uncooked vegetables, salads and unpeeled fruit;
- drink only pasteurized or sterilized milk;
- wash your hands well and regularly, especially after going to the toilet or preparing food or eating (do not share towels);
- use only your own eating utensils, toothbrushes, razors or any other items that could have blood on them.

Your doctor can vaccinate against HAV, either alone or with vaccines against hepatitis B virus (HBV) or typhoid fever. Talk to your doctor at least six weeks before you plan to travel or if you're at high risk of contracting the virus, such as if you:

- are a man who has sex with other men;
- inject heroin or other street drugs;
- work with or near sewage;
- work where hygiene is poor;
- have a chronic liver disease;
- take drugs for haemophilia made from donated blood. Screening donated blood reduces the risk of contracting HAV and other viruses, but a very small risk remains.

Hepatitis B

Infected blood or body fluids transmit HBV. So, you can catch HBV:

- during sex with an infected partner;
- by sharing contaminated equipment to inject street drugs;
- during pregnancy, when an infected mother passes HBV to her unborn child;
- after receiving infected blood transfusions or treatments made from blood;
- by being accidently stabbed with a needle contaminated with infected blood;
- by being tattooed, receiving acupuncture or having body piercing with equipment that has not been sterilized properly.

Several viruses share HBV's routes of transmission, including HCV and HIV, responsible for AIDS. So, taking steps to avoid one virus helps protect you from others.

The course of HBV

Often HBV infection does not initially cause symptoms. Nevertheless, some people experience symptoms such as:

- a flu-like illness, including sore throat, tiredness, joint pains and loss of appetite;
- nausea;
- vomiting;
- abdominal discomfort;
- jaundice.

In around 1 in 20 adults and about 9 in 10 children, HBV continues to replicate in liver cells after any initial symptoms resolve. If the immune system does not clear the virus within six months, doctors regard the person as having chronic HBV. As many people do not experience symptoms, they are unaware that they have chronic HBV. Nevertheless, they remain infectious as well as being at risk of developing cirrhosis and up to 100 times more likely to develop liver cancer.

Treating and preventing HBV

The body naturally produces proteins called inter-ferons, some of which directly attack HBV and bolster the immune system's ability to tackle infected hepato-cytes. Drug companies have also developed therapeutic interferons for several diseases including HBV, HCV and certain cancers. You inject interferon into the layer of fat just under your skin for several months. However, some people – such as those with advanced liver disease – may not be able to receive interferons. Serious side effects are uncommon, although interferons can cause, for example, influenza-like symptoms, depres-sion and fatigue.

Some drugs directly attack HBV. These antivirals do not need to be injected, produce fewer side effects than interferons and are suitable for people with advanced liver disease. However, antivirals do not always work. Furthermore, HBV can mutate, so after a while the antiviral may not work as effectively. Your doctor will help you decide which drug is suitable for you. Check out the information provided by patient groups and discuss the risks and benefits fully.

Vaccination

Discuss vaccination with your doctor if you are one of those at high risk of catching HBV, such as:

- people who inject heroin and other street drugs;
- heterosexual people who change sexual partners frequently;
- men who have sex with men;
- babies born to HBV-positive mothers;
- close family and friends of infected people;
- patients who need blood transfusions or regularly use medicines made from blood;
- people with other liver diseases or chronic kidney disease;
- people travelling to countries where HBV is widespread;
- families adopting children from countries where HBV is common;
- prisoners and people in high-risk occupations, including sex workers, nurses, prison wardens, doctors, dentists and laboratory staff.

Hepatitis C

HCV spreads from contact with blood from an infected person, usually, in the UK, by injecting street drugs. Blood transfusions and products, sex and other members of the same household can also transmit HCV. Many people do not develop symptoms when they catch HCV. However, you may experience for example:

- fatigue
- poor appetite
- weight loss
- depression
- anxiety
- problems with memory and concentration
- pain or discomfort in the abdomen.

Up to 20 per cent of people clear HCV naturally within six months. In the remainder, the course of chronic HCV varies widely:

- Many people don't develop symptoms and remain unaware that they carry HCV. They remain infectious, however.
- At least one-quarter develop cirrhosis within 30–40 years of infection.
- Up to 1 in 25 people with cirrhosis due to HCV develop liver cancer each year.

Doctors cannot yet tell who will develop HCV's serious complications.

Alcohol and HCV

Up to 70 per cent of people infected with HCV abuse alcohol or previously had a drinking problem, while around 30 per cent of people with alcoholic liver disease are infected. Everyone with HCV should ideally avoid alcohol. Even moderate alcohol consumption can hasten cirrhosis in people with HCV. Abstinence may reverse alcohol-related damage, improve the response to treatment and reduce cirrhosis risk.

As there is no vaccine, preventing HCV focuses on good hygiene, such as:

- using disposable sterile needles for body piercing;
- not sharing toothbrushes, razors and other items that could be contaminated with blood;
- covering wounds and cuts with waterproof dressings;
- using undiluted bleach to clean up blood spills.

Interferons and a growing number of antivirals can cure chronic HCV infections in some people. Cure rates with some of the newer combinations may reach 90–100 per cent, provided you take the treatment, which lasts several months. Learn all you can, such as from the websites of patient groups, and discuss the risks and benefits fully with your doctor.

Hepatitis D

An outer coat surrounds each hepatitis virus. Hepatitis D virus (HDV) needs HBV to make its coat. So, for HDV to replicate you also need to be infected with HBV.

HDV worsens your prospects compared to being infected with HBV alone. For example, people infected with HBV and HDV are some 137 times more likely to develop hepatocellular carcinoma (HCC), the most common liver cancer, than those infected with neither virus. HDV commonly spreads by injecting street drugs, sex and within families. Sometimes, interferon may eradicate HDV or normalize liver function tests. As scientists have not developed a vaccine, good hygiene is the best way to avoid HDV.

Hepatitis E

HEV rarely causes chronic infection, but may cause, for example:

- jaundice
- dark brown urine
- pale clay-coloured stools
- tiredness
- fever
- nausea and vomiting
- abdominal pain
- appetite loss.

Symptoms usually develop about 40 days after infection and resolve within one to four weeks.

As most people clear HEV naturally, doctors do not specifically treat the infection. However, pregnant and older people, those with weakened immune systems and people with chronic liver disease might experience more severe symptoms. Indeed, occasionally, HEV rapidly proves fatal, particularly in pregnant women.

HEV spreads from faecal contamination of food and water. So, the tips on page 18 will help prevent HEV. During the illness:

- avoid alcohol;
- do not prepare meals for other people, especially during the first two weeks;
- limit contact with others, especially with pregnant women and people with chronic liver disease.

5

Alcoholic liver disease

Millions of people put their health at risk by drinking too much alcohol. Indeed, alcohol accounts for almost two-fifths of deaths from liver disease, as well as increasing the risk of, for example, heart attacks, strokes and several cancers. Alcohol abuse can also irreconcilably damage families and cause accidents that injure or kill yourself or others. If you know someone who is abusing alcohol, gently and sympathetically advise them to seek help.

A UK unit of alcohol

You should discuss the alcohol consumption that's right for you with your doctor. One unit of alcohol contains 8 g alcohol. So:

- Half a pint of normal strength beer, lager or cider equals one unit.
- One small (100 ml) glass of wine equals one unit.
- A large (175 ml) glass of wine equals two units.
- A single (25 ml) measure of spirits equals one unit.
- One 275 ml bottle of alcopop (5.5 per cent/volume) equals 1.5 units.

An American 'drink' contains 14 g of alcohol or just less than two UK units.

The liver and alcohol

The risk of developing cirrhosis doubles once alcohol consumption exceeds 50 g (about six units) daily and increases approximately fivefold among those drinking more than 100 g a day (about 13 units). Up to about a third of people who drink heavily for several years show alcohol-related hepatitis. Up to a fifth develop cirrhosis. Continuing to drink worsens your prospects:

- Nine out of ten people with compensated cirrhosis (page 8) due to alcohol live for five years if they abstain from drinking.
- Five-year survival declines to less than seven in ten if people with compensated cirrhosis persistently drink.
- At most, three in ten people who continue to drink after developing alcohol-related decompensated liver disease live for five years.

The amount you drink is not the only factor influencing the risk of alcohol-related damage, however. Many people never develop symptomatic liver disease despite years of excessive drinking. But some people develop alcoholic liver disease and cirrhosis even if they have never been dependent on drink. There are several reasons for this. For instance, people who are genetically predisposed to break down alcohol more effectively are less likely to suffer liver damage or become addicted than those with less effective metabolisms. Other people may be genetically 'programmed' to repair damage more efficiently.

Furthermore, some people who abuse alcohol often don't eat healthily, which makes liver damage even more likely. They may replace calories from nutritious food with 'empty' calories from ethanol (the alcohol in alcoholic drinks) or not eat sufficient vitamins A, C, E, folic acid (vitamin B_9), thiamine (vitamin B_1) and pyridoxine (vitamin B_6).

Am I drinking excessively?

If you get so drunk that you can't recall how much you drank, you almost certainly have a problem. Your drinking pattern offers another clue. Most people vary their drinking pattern. People who abuse alcohol tend to drink more regularly, partly to stave off withdrawal symptoms, which can include shakes, insomnia, agitation, depression and even fits.

In addition, if you answer yes to two or more of the CAGE questions you may have an alcohol problem:

C: Have you ever felt you should cut down on your drinking?

A: Have people ever annoyed you by criticizing your drinking?

G: Have you ever felt bad or guilty about your drinking?

E: Eye opener: Have you ever had a drink first thing in the morning to steady your nerves or to get rid of a hangover?

The Alcohol Use Disorders Identification Test (AUDIT) questionnaire (<www.patient.co.uk/doctor/alcohol-use-disorders-identification-test-audit>) offers a more comprehensive assessment of alcohol use. Your doctor might also use the Fast Alcohol Screening Test (FAST; <www.nhs.uk/Conditions/Alcohol-misuse/Pages/diagnosis.aspx>) and Severity of Alcohol Dependence Questionnaire (SADQ; <www.drinksafely.soton.ac.uk/SADQ/>).

Cutting down your drinking

If you suspect you might be drinking excessively, keep a diary for about a month and note how much you drink and when (places and circumstances, such as when you're feeling down, stressed or with certain people). The average adult drinker underestimates consumption by the equivalent of a bottle of wine each week. So, don't guess, and be honest.

Then set a goal. Some people will need to abstain. Others find that they can cut back to within the recommended limit – but should remain alert for changes in their drinking habits. If you have liver disease or any other health problem, you should follow your doctor's advice, which may differ from the general safe drinking limits.

Tricks to reduce consumption

To reduce your alcohol consumption:

- Favour drinks with a lower alcohol content.
- Replace large wine glasses with smaller ones.
- Buy a measure so you can tell how many units of spirit you're pouring.
- Only drink alcohol with a meal.
- Alternate alcoholic beverages with water or soft drinks.
- Drink spritzers and shandies rather than wine and beer.
- Add more water or mixers to spirits.
- Have dry days each week.
- Find a hobby that does not involve drinking.
- Spend at least some of the money you save on something for yourself.

Some people pick a day to stop or dramatically cut down. Others gradually reduce the amount they drink. (Keep a diary if you're slowly cutting down to make sure you don't slip back.) Even if you plan to return to drinking safe levels of alcohol, it's worth 'drying out' for at least a month and taking milk thistle (page 61) to give your liver a chance to recover.

Deciding whether to tell your family, friends and colleagues that you're cutting down can be difficult. Some offer advice and support, especially if they have expressed concern about your drinking. But they may underestimate the strength of alcohol addiction and not be as understanding if you slip back. However, some people may feel that you are challenging their drinking habits, and may prove hostile or condescending, especially if some of your social or work life revolves around drinking. Counselling (see the British Association for Counselling and Psychotherapy; <www.bacp.co.uk>) can help you understand why you drink, how to cut down and the best way to deal with difficult situations. You could also change your social life or tell some white lies to explain your abstinence.

Alcohol services are available on the NHS. Doctors can prescribe drugs to help you deal with cravings. Support groups (e.g. Alcoholics Anonymous; <www.alcoholics-anonymous.org.uk/>) help many people. So, there is plenty of help available. The most difficult step is accepting that you need help and, if you can't cut back alone, asking for assistance.

6

Non-alcoholic liver disease

Walk down any high street and it's clear from the double chins, sagging bottoms and bulging waistbands that too many of us carry too much weight. Being overweight or obese causes or contributes to numerous serious conditions, including heart disease, diabetes and some cancers. As your weight rises, fat gradually deposits in your liver causing non-alcoholic fatty liver disease (NAFLD), which is the leading cause of chronic liver damage in Western countries. Almost all (95 per cent) obese people and three-quarters of people with diabetes have NAFLD.

A healthy liver contains very little or no fat. Doctors generally diagnose NAFLD when a liver contains more than 5 per cent fat (on average 60–75 g) after excluding other causes, such as alcohol, viral hepatitis or certain medicines. Initially at least, a fatty liver, which doctors call 'steatosis', does not cause symptoms.

Fat deposits can, however, trigger inflammation in and around the liver cells – so-called non-alcoholic steatohepatitis (NASH) – causing swelling of, and discomfort or pain around, the liver. Over time, NASH can progress to cirrhosis, irreversible liver damage and liver cancer. Doctors often detect NAFLD when they feel an enlarged liver or find mild changes in LFTs (page 16). Doctors use a liver biopsy to distinguish NASH from simple steatosis.

Treating NAFLD

The decline from steatosis, which can end in cancer, is not inevitable. Doctors have yet to find a medicine that treats NAFLD. So, doctors generally suggest that patients:

- increase exercise, which burns fat;
- eat a low-fat, healthy diet;
- avoid alcohol;
- avoid unnecessary medicines;
- lose weight, which stops or reverses liver damage in NASH patients: losing 4.5–6.8 kg (10–15 lb) often returns liver function tests to normal.

Tackling free radicals

A slice of apple left exposed to the air turns brown, caused by a group of chemicals called free radicals. Free radicals also contribute to liver damage in NASH. Indeed, people with NASH tend to have low blood levels of vitamin E and certain carotenoids (yellow, orange and red pigments in plants) that mop up tissue-damaging free radicals. So, it's a good idea to eat foods rich in carotenoids and vitamin E. You could also think about a supplement – after speaking to your doctor first.

7

Liver cancer

Liver cancer accounts for about 1 in every 100 malignancies in the UK. Tragically, most of those affected face a bleak future. According to Cancer Research UK, only three in every ten people with liver cancer survive for a year or more after diagnosis. However, you can reduce your risk of developing liver cancer.

Cancer: cells out of control

Normally cells divide, under tight control, to replace old and damaged tissue. Damaged cells that do not die or new cells that form when they should not can create a swelling, called a tumour.

Some accumulations of cells create 'benign' tumours that are not cancerous and, usually, do not recur after surgery. Benign tumours in the liver include:

- *Haemangiomas* These are the most common benign liver tumour, start in blood vessels and usually don't need treatment. A surgeon may remove tumours that start bleeding.
- *Hepatic adenomas* These begin in hepatocytes and can cause pain, create a lump in the abdomen or bleed. As hepatic adenomas can rupture, causing severe blood loss, and there is a small risk they could transform into a cancer, a doctor may suggest removal.

- *Focal nodular hyperplasia (FNH)* This a mass of several different types of cell, including hepatocytes and bile duct cells. Doctors often find distinguishing FNH from liver cancers difficult and may remove the growth as a precaution.

Cancerous cells divide uncontrollably, invade surrounding healthy tissue and, in time, spread to other parts of the body (metastasis). Most cancers are named after their site of origin:

- Primary hepatocellular carcinomas (HCCs) develop in hepatocytes.
- Cholangiocarcinomas arise in bile ducts.
- Angiosarcomas affect blood vessels in the liver.

Secondary liver cancers spread from a primary malignancy in, for example, the breast, lung or bowel. Doctors classify the secondary liver malignancies based on the site of the primary cancer: for example, liver metastases of breast cancer.

Risk factors for liver cancer

- *Chronic liver disease* Between 70 and 90 per cent of HCCs develop in people with chronic liver disease. For example, one-third of people with cirrhosis eventually develop HCC.
- *Infections* HBV and HCV cause about half and a third respectively of HCCs worldwide.
- *Aflatoxin* is a poison produced by a fungus that grows on mouldy peanuts, wheat, soya, corn, rice and so on, and is especially common in parts of Africa and Asia. Aflatoxin increases the risk of liver cancer only if people eat food colonized by the fungus over a long time or if they are infected with HBV.

- *Alcohol abuse* causes around 1 in 20 avoidable liver cancers in women and approximately 1 in 10 in men.
- *Betel quid* Chewing betel quid as a stimulant and relaxant is relatively common across the Indian subcontinent, Asia and parts of the Pacific, but may more than treble the risk of liver cancer. People infected with HBV who chewed betel were five times more likely to develop liver cancer than those with the virus alone. Chewing betel quid almost doubled the risk of liver cancer in people with HCV.
- *Diabetes* The risk that a person with diabetes and HBV or HCV will develop HCC is around 100 times higher than in infected people who are neither obese nor diabetic.
- *Obesity* Obese people are two to three times more likely to develop HCC than their thinner counterparts. Obesity also increases the likelihood that people infected with HBV or HCV will develop HCC.
- *Smoking* Carcinogens in cigarette smoke can enter the blood and trigger liver cancer.
- *Age* Liver cancer becomes more common with advancing age, partly because the cancer usually takes many years to develop.
- *Family history* Having a parent who develops liver cancer increases the risk of HCC more than sixfold. Genetic factors may influence the risk. You may also share environmental risk factors.
- *Sex* Around two-thirds of liver cancers occur in men, probably because of differences in risk factors (such as alcohol consumption).

You can't do much about some of these risk factors. But they rarely act in isolation. So, if you quit smoking and

Table 3 Possible symptoms of primary liver cancer

Marked weight loss (such as losing 1 stone (6.4 kg) if you weigh 11 stone or 70 kg) that cannot be explained (such as by dieting)

Losing your appetite for a few weeks

Vomiting

Feeling full or bloated after eating a relatively small meal

Pain, discomfort or swelling in your tummy (abdomen)

Yellow-tinged skin (jaundice), dark brownish urine, pale clay-coloured faeces

Itching

Sudden worsening of your health if you have chronic hepatitis or cirrhosis

High temperature or sweating

Source: Adapted from Cancer Research UK

reduce your alcohol consumption, you'll improve your chances of avoiding liver cancer whatever your age, family history or sex.

Detecting liver cancer

If you develop any symptom in Table 3 you should see your doctor as soon as possible – even if you've already been diagnosed with chronic liver disease. Doctors will check whether you have liver cancer using, for example:

- *Biopsy*, which is examined and tested for cancer's hallmark changes. However, biopsies may miss 30 per cent of HCCs. Between 1 and 5 per cent of biopsies allow the cancer to spread to another part of the liver.

- *Blood tests*, including liver function tests and measuring blood levels of a chemical called alpha-fetoprotein. Normally, foetuses produce alpha-fetoprotein. However, blood levels increase in about 60 per cent of people with liver cancer.
- *Imaging* By looking for changes between visits, ultrasonography can detect around 90 per cent of tumours before symptoms develop. Ultrasonography is more likely to miss tumours that are already present at the first visit because the doctors do not have a previous image. Overall, ultrasonography detects around 60–80 per cent of liver cancers. Doctors may suggest using CT or MRI to detect the cancer.

Treating liver cancer

Doctors detect about one malignancy in ten early enough for surgery and liver transplantation to markedly improve chances of a cure. More commonly, drugs and surgery lengthen survival rather than cure. So, see your doctor as soon as possible if you think there is anything wrong. Discussing risks and benefits can help you and your cancer team decide the best approach for you.

Surgery

Surgery to cut away the cancer (hepatic resection) is the treatment of choice for HCC without marked cirrhosis, especially if you have a single tumour. In some people with cirrhosis, however, resection can result in liver failure.

Liver transplant

Liver transplants raise the prospect of a cure – 75 per cent of recipients are still alive at least five years after receiving their new organ. However, there are too few donated organs to meet demand and you'll need to take powerful drugs to reduce the risk that you'll reject your new liver. These drugs can cause potentially serious side effects.

Ablation

Doctors may try to destroy early HCC by injecting a chemical into the cancer, using radio waves, microwaves, lasers or extreme cold. Ablation using ethanol and radio waves can destroy almost all HCCs that are smaller than 2 cm. Ablation is less effective against larger tumours and is not suitable for cancers near major blood vessels, bile ducts, the bowel, heart or other critical organs.

Chemoembolization

Blocking the blood vessels supplying the cancer – using, for example, tiny spheres – will starve the cancer of oxygen and nutrients and so limit growth. The spheres also slowly release a cancer drug – attacking the malignancy on two fronts. However, cancers can grow blood vessels that bypass the block. Chemoembolization does not attack small cancers that have not yet produced blood vessels, but which could develop into large tumours.

Drugs for liver cancer

A growing number of drugs are showing promise for advanced liver cancer. Our rapidly advancing understanding of liver cancer's causes, development and spread means that several more will probably reach the clinic over the next few years. Ask your oncologist about these options and taking part in a clinical study of a new treatment for liver cancer.

8

Other diseases of the liver

Alcohol abuse, viruses and obesity cause most liver diseases. However, more than 100 ailments can damage the liver, as the following examples illustrate. Try the National Digestive Diseases Information Clearinghouse (<digestive.niddk.nih.gov>) and the British Liver Trust (<www.britishlivertrust.org.uk>) for more information.

Porphyria

The body makes haem, the red pigment in blood and part of the protein that carries oxygen, in seven steps, each controlled by a different enzyme. Porphyria arises when one of these enzymes (usually because of an abnormal gene) does not work properly. Levels of the preceding protein rise, which causes the symptoms. Heavy alcohol consumption, iron supplements, certain drugs and liver infections can trigger a form of the disease called porphyria cutanea tarda. To learn more, contact the British Porphyria Association (<www.porphyria.org.uk/>).

Acute attacks

Four of the seven subtypes of porphyria cause sudden (acute) attacks. For instance, about one person in five with acute intermittent porphyria and variegate porphyria develops acute attacks characterized by:

- severe pain in the stomach, back or thighs;

- nausea, vomiting and constipation;
- red, brown or purple urine (the sample may change colour when stored);
- low levels of salt or sodium in the blood;
- rapid pulse and dangerously high blood pressure (hypertension);
- loss of movement in the arms or legs.

Some people experience only one or two acute attacks, which may be triggered by, for example, alcohol and certain drugs. Porphyrins can also accumulate in the skin. In five forms of porphyria, when light hits skin laden with porphyrins, the reaction damages the surrounding tissues. As a result, the skin can blister, burn easily in the sun and, in some cases, scar. Treatment largely focuses on avoiding triggers (such as sun exposure and certain medicines).

Haemochromatosis

Iron is vital for several biological reactions, including allowing red blood cells to carry oxygen. People with hereditary (primary) haemochromatosis are born with a genetic defect that leads to excessive levels of iron in their body, including the liver. Some patients with alcoholic liver disease, NASH or HCV infection also accumulate iron ('secondary haemochromatosis').

Initially, doctors treat haemochromatosis by draining about 500 ml of blood (phlebotomy) every week until iron levels normalize. This can take a year. Doctors then remove blood every two to four weeks to keep iron at safe levels. If phlebotomy is not appropriate, doctors may use a drug that removes iron from blood. Contact the Haemochromatosis Society UK (<www.haemochromatosis.org.uk>).

Wilson's disease

Normally, the liver stores the small amounts of copper that the body needs to remain healthy and excretes any excess in bile. But about 1 in 40,000 people develop Wilson's disease, a genetic disorder that prevents the body from removing excess copper.

The gradual accumulation of copper damages the liver, brain and spinal cord, and other organs. This potentially causes debilitating symptoms, including:

- altered behaviour
- ascites (page 11)
- jaundice
- Kayser–Fleischer rings (a rusty-brown ring around the iris and the rim of the cornea)
- liver failure
- problems with speech and swallowing
- problems with physical coordination, and tremors or uncontrolled movements.

Symptoms usually appear between 5 and 35 years of age, but can emerge at almost any age.

Treatment aims to remove excess copper, reduce copper intake and treat any damage. Some drugs release stores of copper from organs into the bloodstream; the copper is then excreted. Other medicines block absorption of copper from food. So, people with Wilson's disease need to avoid shellfish or liver. They can eat mushrooms, broccoli, nuts and chocolate in moderation once symptoms abate.

Alpha-1 antitrypsin deficiency

Patients with alpha-1 antitrypsin (A1AT) deficiency, another inherited condition, lack an important protein made by the liver. In the lungs, for example, an enzyme (neutrophil elastase) destroys damaged or old lung cells, foreign particles and bacteria. A1AT prevents neutrophil elastase from damaging healthy tissue. In A1AT deficiency, high levels of neutrophil elastase cause a potentially debilitating lung disease called emphysema, which makes breathing difficult.

A1AT deficiency can cause liver disease. So, people with A1AT deficiency should:

- not drink alcohol;
- when possible, avoid medicines that may harm the liver;
- eat plenty of fresh fruit and vegetables;
- take exercise to help boost the immune system;
- avoid tobacco smoke and pollution. A1AT-deficient lungs are especially vulnerable to damage by pollution and smoking.

Autoimmune diseases

Autoimmune hepatitis follows an attack on liver cells by the body's immune system, which causes inflammation and, over time, liver damage. Autoimmune hepatitis is often relatively serious and, if not treated with drugs that dampen the immune response, can end in cirrhosis and liver failure.

Primary biliary cirrhosis

During primary biliary cirrhosis (PBC), an autoimmune attack slowly destroys bile ducts. So, bile leaks from the ducts and damages surrounding liver cells. As the liver can initially compensate, PBC may not cause symptoms at first. But, over many years, the damage causes cirrhosis. Doctors can use several drugs to treat PBC; occasionally, patients need a liver transplant. Many people find that they need to adapt their lifestyle to cope with the fatigue, which is common in PBC. Eating regular small meals often ensures that bile has some food to digest, which spares your liver.

Primary sclerosing cholangitis

In primary sclerosing cholangitis, scar tissue narrows and then completely blocks bile ducts. The resulting hepatic damage causes the typical symptoms of liver disease (such as itching, jaundice and abdominal pain) and, in some patients, cirrhosis, portal hypertension and liver failure. Currently, there is no cure or treatment that slows progression. Some people eventually need liver transplants.

Gallstones

Gallstones are pebble-like deposits inside the gall bladder, ranging in size from a grain of sand to a golf ball. Cholesterol (or, less commonly, bilirubin released during the destruction of old red blood cells) forms stones. Several factors increase the risk of developing gallstones (Table 4 overleaf).

Doctors often diagnose gallstones on an X-ray, during surgery and so on. Large stones blocking the bile duct can cause pain in the middle to right upper abdomen (biliary colic). Other people develop fever, jaundice, pass clay-coloured stools or experience

Table 4 Factors that may increase the risk of developing gallstones

Factor	Explanation
Being female	Oestrogen during pregnancy and from hormone replacement therapy and the pill seem to increase the risk. Overall, two women develop gallstones for each man with the condition.
Diabetes	People with diabetes often show high levels of triglycerides (page 4), which increases the likelihood of developing gallstones.
Genetics	Gallstones seem to run in families.
Weight	Even being moderately overweight seems to increase the risk. The link between obesity and gallstones seems to be especially strong in women. But avoid rapid weight loss ('crash diets'), which can increase your risk of developing gallstones.
Unhealthy diet	A diet high in fat and cholesterol and low in fibre increases the amount of cholesterol in bile and can stop the gall bladder from emptying properly.
Age	You are more likely to develop gallstones once you are over 60 years of age.
Cholesterol-lowering drugs	These may increase the amount removed in the bile.

nausea and vomiting. See your GP if you develop any of these symptoms.

Usually, gallstones that don't cause symptoms do not need surgery. However, people who develop symptoms will probably need surgery, although doctors can also prescribe medicines that dissolve gallstones made from cholesterol. (These may take two years or more to work.) Another approach uses sound waves to break up the stones. However, in both cases, gallstones may form again when treatment ends.

Medicines that harm the liver

The liver breaks down many medicines and other chemicals. Usually, the liver makes the medicine less active. But some drugs do not work unless they are first converted by the liver.

Some drugs trigger the liver to produce larger quantities of one or more enzyme – so-called inducers. If you take an inducer with another drug broken down by the same enzyme, the liver may remove the second drug too quickly. So, the medicine may not work as well as if you didn't take the inducer.

Other drugs inhibit the drug-metabolizing enzyme. Taking a drug metabolized by an enzyme along with an inhibitor of the same enzyme could allow blood levels of medicine to rise, potentially causing serious side effects. Such interactions are one reason why you should let your doctor and pharmacist know when you are using herbal remedies and other medicines, whether prescribed or bought from a pharmacist or a health shop. You can also check the summary of product characteristics (<www.medicines.org.uk/emc>) for potential interactions with foods and drugs.

Chronic liver disease can undermine your ability to metabolize certain drugs. So, your doctor may lower the dose of some drugs to compensate. Furthermore, numerous drugs can damage the liver, including some medicines used to lower cholesterol, certain antifungals and several painkillers, including paracetamol.

So, if you have liver disease, don't buy painkillers or other medicines without checking with a pharmacist or doctor first. Your doctor may suggest liver function tests before you start taking a medicine and regularly during treatment. You may stop treatment if liver function tests are abnormal. You should tell your doctor if you develop symptoms that might indicate liver damage, such as jaundice, weight loss, nausea, itching, fatigue and pain in the right upper abdomen.

9

Diet and liver disease

The typical modern Western diet produces too much energy. If you do not burn this energy off, the body stores the surplus. So, we gain weight, especially around our middle (central obesity), which contributes to NAFLD and numerous other diseases.

So everyone, especially people with liver disease, should eat a healthy, balanced diet. Changing your diet can seem daunting. But many people find that it takes only a month or so of eating – or not eating – a food to form a habit, such as not needing as much salt. Furthermore, most complementary healers emphasize the importance of a healthy diet as a cornerstone of detox.

Salt

High salt levels damage cells. So, your body retains fluid to dilute the salt. But retaining fluid increases blood pressure and makes it more likely you'll develop hypertension, which can lead to strokes and heart disease.

Unfortunately, many people in the UK eat too much salt: the recommended intake for healthy adults is 6 g of salt a day – about a teaspoon. But follow your doctor's advice: some people with liver disease and certain other conditions need to consume even less. People with cirrhosis tend to retain salt, for example.

Watch, in particular, for hidden salt. It's easy to tell that some snacks are salty. But many foods – including some soups, bread, biscuits and breakfast cereals – contain 'hidden' salt, so your taste buds will not set the alarm bells ringing. So, always read the label. Try to choose meals and sandwiches with less than 1.25 g salt or individual foods, such as soups and sauces, with less than 0.75 g per serving. In addition:

- Add as little salt as you can during baking and cooking.
- Banish the salt cellar from the table.
- Ask restaurants and take-aways for 'no salt'.
- Look for low-salt ketchup, pickles, mustard, yeast extract, stock cubes and so on.
- Try flavouring with herbs, spices, chopped chillies and lime or lemon juice.

Some labels list sodium, rather than salt. Chemically, table salt is sodium chloride. To convert sodium to salt, multiply by 2.5. So, 0.4 g of sodium is 1 g of salt. You can convert salt to sodium by dividing by 2.5.

Protein

Protein's numerous essential biological roles include:

- helping the liver and other tissues repair and regenerate;
- forming specialized proteins, such as enzymes;
- forming the scaffold that supports the cell;
- making antibodies, which help fight infections.

A liver damaged by, for example, cirrhosis may not use protein effectively, potentially leading to muscle wasting and osteoporosis. As a result, people with liver disease may need to eat plenty of protein, such as 1.0–1.5 g a day for each kilogram of body weight. Your doctor or dietician will tell you how much.

Fish and omega-3 fatty acids

Few plants survive inside the Arctic Circle. So, the traditional diet of First Nation Arctic people consists almost entirely of meat. Yet they seem to be less vulnerable to several ailments, including diabetes, heart disease, arthritis and asthma, than people in industrialized countries.

So, what's their secret? The traditional diets of First Nation Arctic people are packed with fish and animals that, in turn, eat marine life. This means that they eat large amounts of fish oils (called n-3, or omega-3, polyunsaturated fatty acids; PUFAs) that have several important health benefits, including:

- reducing inflammation (which increases in many liver diseases);
- boosting levels of the healthy fat (HDL) in blood;
- cutting triglyceride (page 4) levels, the main fat that accumulates in the liver and a leading cause of steatosis and heart disease;
- lowering blood pressure;
- reducing steatosis (page 30);
- reducing the risk of heart disease and keeping your joints healthy;
- contributing to memory, intellectual performance and healthy vision.

Omega-3 fatty acids – specifically docosahexaenoic acid (DHA) and eicosapentaenoic acid (EPA) – seem to be responsible for most of these benefits. We can make omega-3 fatty acids from green leafy vegetables, nuts, seeds and their oils. But it's a slow process. So, it's a good idea to boost levels by eating fish and seafood high in omega-3 fatty acids.

Adults and children over 12 years of age should eat two portions of fish per week (a portion is about 140 g after cooking). One of these should be an oily fish. If you're eating canned fish, check the label to make sure processing has not depleted the omega-3 oils.

If at first you don't like the taste, try some different fish and a few recipes. If you really can't stomach fish try a supplement – but speak to your doctor first. If, for example, like many people with NAFLD you have diabetes, you may need to avoid omega-3 supplements, which might increase blood sugar levels.

Vegetables, fruit and fibre

A diet that's low in fruit and vegetables can contribute to liver disease. For example, NASH patients tend to

Types of fibre

Fibre (roughage) is the part of plants we cannot digest. There are two main types:

- Insoluble fibre remains largely intact as it moves through your digestive system, but makes defaecation easier.
- Soluble fibre dissolves in the water in the gut forming a gel, which soaks up fats. So, you absorb less fat, which lowers cholesterol levels. Soluble fibre also releases sugar slowly, producing steadier blood levels after you eat. This can help stave off hunger pangs and so helps you lose weight.

have lower levels of certain carotenoids (page 31). On the other hand, a high-fibre diet helps the regular bowel movements that may help remove toxins from the body and reduce the amount of toxins absorbed from foods.

Whole grains are an especially good source of fibre. Grains – the seeds of cereals such as wheat, rye, barley, oats and rice – have three layers:

- Bran, the outer layer, is rich in fibre and packed with nutrients.
- The germ develops into a new plant and is packed with nutrients. Wheat germ, for example, contains high levels of vitamin E, folate (folic acid), zinc, magnesium and other vitamins and minerals.
- The central area (endosperm) is largely starch, which provides the energy the germ needs to develop into a new plant.

Many food manufacturers strip off the bran and germ, which removes up to 75 per cent of the nutritional value. So eat more foods with 'whole' in front of the grain's name – such as wholewheat pasta, wholegrain bread and whole oats.

Five portions of fruit and vegetables

Fruit and vegetables are rich in vitamins, minerals and fibre. So, everyone – not just people with chronic liver disease – should eat at least five portions of fruit and vegetables a day. A portion weighs about 80 g: one medium-sized fruit (banana, apple, pear, orange); a slice of a large fruit (melon, pineapple, mango); or three heaped tablespoons of vegetables or pulses.

Many detox diets emphasize eating raw fruit and vegetables. Certainly, cooking can leach nutrients from fruits and vegetables. If you cook, use a small amount of unsalted water for the shortest time you can, lightly steaming or stir-frying. Scrub rather than peel potatoes, carrots and so on: the skin is rich in nutrients.

Drinking smoothies and soups also boosts your intake of fruit and vegetables. However, some commercial smoothies contain extra sugar, honey, yoghurt or milk, while vegetable soups may contain added salt. So, check the label.

Finally, seeds, nuts and legumes are an excellent source of fibre and other nutrients. But seeds are relatively high in calories. Legumes are a cheap source of protein, are high in fibre and help control levels of fats in the blood. Vegetarian cookbooks are full of ideas to help boost your bean consumption. You can add beans to bulk up stews to cut down on meat.

Eating to lose weight

Weight is not a very good guide to your risk of developing NAFLD, gallstones and other conditions linked to excess body fat. Weighing 14 stone (89 kg) is fine if you're 6 feet 5 inches (1.96 m). But you would be seriously obese if you were 5 feet 6 inches (1.68 m). Body mass index (BMI; <www.nhs.uk/tools/pages/healthy-weightcalculator.aspx>) tells you whether you're overweight or obese based your height and weight.

- Keep your BMI between 18.5 and 24.9 kg/m². Below this and you're dangerously underweight.
- A BMI between 25.0 and 29.9 kg/m² suggests that you are overweight.
- You're probably obese if your BMI exceeds 30.0 kg/m².

BMI is usually a good guide, but may overestimate

Table 5 Waist sizes linked to an increased risk to your health

Group	Health at risk	Health at high risk
Men	Over 94 cm (37 inches)	Over 102 cm (40 inches)
Women	Over 80 cm (32 inches)	Over 88 cm (35 inches)
South Asian men		Over 90 cm (36 inches)
South Asian women		Over 80 cm (32 inches)

Source: Adapted from the British Heart Foundation

body fat in athletes, body-builders and other muscular people. On the other hand, BMI may underestimate body fat in older persons and people who have lost muscle, which can be a symptom of chronic liver disease. Doctors and gyms can use a monitor to check your body fat. However, abdominal obesity damages your health more than fat elsewhere, especially in people of South Asian descent (Table 5).

Unfortunately, losing weight is not easy: millions of years of evolution drive us to consume food in times of feast to help us survive famine. And you can't stop eating as you can quit smoking or drinking excessively. Indeed, crash diets can cause the liver to release more cholesterol into bile and mean the gall bladder does not empty properly, which increases your risk of gall-stones. So:

- Take a long-term view. You'll lose weight more quickly in the first few weeks as you burn off the glycogen stores in your liver (page 4) before you start to lose fat.
- Keep a diary of everything that you eat and drink

for a couple of weeks. You'll see where you pile on calories – the odd biscuit, extra glass of wine or full-fat latte – and if you're eating fatty or high-salt food without realizing.

- Set specific goals, such as to lose 2 stone (13 kg) by Christmas. Eating between 500 and 1,000 calories less each day can reduce weight by between 0.5 and 1.0 kg each week.
- Think about how you tried to lose weight in the past. What techniques and diets worked? Did a support group help?
- Don't let a slip-up derail your diet. Try to identify why you indulged. Was it a particular occasion? Do you comfort eat? Then develop strategies to stop future slip-ups.
- Begin your diet when you're at home over a weekend or a holiday and you don't have a celebration (such as Christmas or a birthday) planned.

If all this fails, try talking to your GP or pharmacist. (Make sure he or she knows you have chronic liver disease and any other ailments.) Some medicines may help kick-start your weight loss, but none offers a magic cure. You'll still need to change your lifestyle. However, they may help put you on the right course towards weight loss.

Boost your exercise

Exercise also helps you lose weight and has several other health benefits. Ideally, be moderately active for at least 30 minutes on at least five days – and ideally every day – a week. It does not all have to be in one go. You could exercise for 15 minutes twice a day. Exercise until you are breathing harder than usual, but not so hard that you can't hold a conversation. You should feel that your heart is beating faster than usual and you've begun to sweat. If you experience chest pain, or feel faint or otherwise unwell, stop exercising and see your doctor.

If you've been exercising regularly for a year, you'll lose about half your cardiovascular fitness in just three months if you stop. So, find a type of exercise that suits you and that fits into your lifestyle. If you don't like exercise classes and you join a gym some distance from home or work, you're less likely to stick to the programme. And try to integrate exercise into your everyday life:

- Walk to the local shops.
- Ride a bike to work.
- Park a 15-minute walk from your place of work.
- Get off the bus, tube or metro one or two stops early.
- Use the stairs instead of the lift.
- Clean the house regularly.
- Wash your car by hand.
- Grow your own vegetables.
- Walk around country parks and nature reserves in your area.

Diet, dehydration and detox

A healthy, balanced diet is the foundation of most detox regimens. Some detox practitioners suggest eating fruit and vegetables exclusively (and often raw) for anything between a day and a week. Almost all detox diets eliminate sugar, white flour, additives and so on and suggest drinking plenty of water and herbal teas. Complementary therapists claim this helps flush toxins out of your body.

Scientific studies show that even mild dehydration can cause, for example:

- poor concentration
- poor memory
- increased tension or anxiety
- fatigue
- headache.

In general, adults should drink 1.2 litres of water (six to eight glasses) a day. Drink more during exercise or hot weather, if you feel lightheaded, pass dark-coloured urine, haven't passed urine within six hours or feel thirsty for long periods. See your doctor if you still regularly feel thirsty. Excessive thirst can be a sign of diabetes.

10

Using herbs to cleanse the liver

Humanity has long sought treatments for liver diseases. Traditional British herbalists used several herbal liver tonics, including agrimony (once called liverwort), dandelion, rosemary and sage. Ancient Egyptians treated liver problems with chicory mixed with wine. And a growing number of scientific studies suggest that some herbs, such as milk thistle, protect the liver. On the other hand, some herbal remedies can damage the liver (Table 6 overleaf). You can use the Livertox site (<http://livertox.nih.gov>) to check if studies have linked a herb or drug to liver problems.

Detoxification and 'cleanses'

According to detox's advocates, if our liver or gastro-intestinal tract performs poorly, increasing levels of toxins cause, for example, poor complexion, lethargy, mental slowness, gastrointestinal upsets, muscular aches and pains, and headaches. So, detox uses a mix of approaches – diets, herbs, vitamins, colonic irrigation, liver flushes and cleanses, enemas, saunas and homeopathic remedies – to remove 'toxins'.

Some alternative healers believe that detox drives out toxins accumulated over decades in the liver and other tissues. This, they suggest, can produce a

Table 6 Herbs that may be linked to liver damage

Common name	Latin name	Comments
Amanita mushrooms	Species of *Amanita*, such as *A. muscaria*	Known as fly agaric
Chaparral	*Larrea tridentata*	A native American herb
Comfrey	Species of *Symphytum*, such as *S. officinale*	Traditionally used to help bones heal
Echinacea	Species of *Echinacea*	Sometimes used to boost the immune system and help fight colds
Germander	Species of *Teucrium*	Traditionally used for gout and as a tonic
Jin bu huan		A traditional Chinese herbal sedative and analgesic that can contain several herbs; a number of traditional Chinese herbal remedies have been linked to liver damage
Kava kava	*Piper methysticum*	Used to treat anxiety; sale is banned in the UK
Mistletoe	*Viscum album* and related species	Apart from the traditional use at Christmas, doctors in some European countries prescribe mistletoe extracts as a cancer treatment

Common name	Latin name	Comments
Pennyroyal	*Mentha pulegium*	Traditionally used for menstrual problems, abortions, upset stomach, etc.
Senna	*Senna alexandrina* (sometimes called *Cassia officinalis*)	Widely used as a laxative
Valerian	*Valeriana officinalis*	Used in some 'natural' remedies for sleep disorders; check the label

detox 'crisis', characterized by, for example, headaches, fatigue and abdominal discomfort. The healer and the person undergoing detox can mistake adverse events for a crisis. So, be careful if you experience anything unexpected during detox.

Critics note that very little scientific evidence supports detox. Nevertheless, studies suggest that air pollution (a cocktail of toxic chemicals) increases the risk of death from diseases of the heart and blood vessels, and can exacerbate asthma and undermine how well your lungs work. The health risks of excessive levels of heavy metals such as lead, mercury and copper are beyond debate. So, the link between ill-health and toxins does not seem that unlikely.

If you want to detox, check with your doctor first, especially if you have liver disease or any other medical condition. Consult a registered practitioner, such as one recognized by the General Regulatory Council for Complementary Therapies (<www.grcct.org/>). Read up on the approach and make sure you understand the risks and benefits.

Check carefully before you flush

A liver flush might involving drinking juices, Epsom salts, some oils, certain herbs or preparations of enzymes. You'll flush for a couple days and pass several bowel movements. Some people experience nausea, vomiting and diarrhoea. In addition, oily preparations may contract the gall bladder and any stones could lodge in the duct. As we've seen, some herbs can damage the liver (Table 6). So you need to be careful about any flush, the practitioner suggesting the cleanse and the components of the formulation. Don't buy any conventional medicine, supplement or alternative formulation over the internet unless you are absolutely sure the site is reputable.

Herbs for hepatic health

A growing body of scientific evidence suggests that certain herbs alleviate liver disease and bolster hepatic health. It's best to see a qualified practitioner, such as a medical herbalist (National Institute of Medical Herbalists; <www.nimh.org.uk>), and speak to your doctor before using any herbal treatment for liver disease or another condition. Some herbs can interfere with conventional medicines. So, tell your pharmacist, GP or nurse that you are also taking a herbal medicine. Similarly, tell your medical herbalist about any conventional drugs you're taking. Stop taking the herb if you feel unwell, and if you feel that you are not benefiting after three months or so, or you develop any changes that could be side effects, stop taking the formulation and see your practitioner.

Ayurvedic medicine

Indian Ayurvedic medicine, which is among the world's longest-established healing traditions, uses about 90 herbs in some 300 preparations for jaundice and chronic liver disease alone, including the arjun tree and katuka.

In experiments using mice, extracts of the arjun tree's smooth grey bark seem to protect the liver from damage by carbon tetrachloride, one of the most potent hepatic toxins. Traditional Indian healers use katuka to treat jaundice. Again, katuka seems to protect the liver against damage from carbon tetrachloride, paracetamol and some other toxins. Contact the Ayurvedic Practitioners Association (<apa.uk.com>) or the British Association of Accredited Ayurvedic Practitioners (<www.britayurpractitioners.com>).

Milk thistle

Milk thistle (*Silybum marianum*), a member of the same botanical family as daisies and sunflowers, grows wild across southern Europe, southern Russia, Asia Minor and North Africa. Since antiquity, European healers have used milk thistle to treat liver and gall bladder disorders, including hepatitis, cirrhosis and jaundice, as well as protecting against chemical poisons, snake bites, insect stings, mushroom poisoning and alcohol.

Scientists now know that milk thistle contains several active chemicals. The extract of milk thistle used commonly, called silymarin, contains four chemicals, including silibinin (silybin). Experimental studies suggest that silibinin alone and silymarin:

- protect the liver from toxins;

- mop up tissue-damaging free radicals;
- counter inflammation;
- reduce fibrosis (scarring);
- increase protein production, which may help repair damaged hepatocytes;
- reduce the absorption of some poisons;
- may directly kill cancer cells;
- augment some conventional cancer treatments.

In clinical trials, silymarin seems to treat poisoning with the aptly named Death Cap mushroom. In alcoholic liver disease, silymarin seems to counter abnormal liver function tests, normalize damaged areas of the liver and slow the progression of fibrosis. Silymarin does not inhibit replication of viruses responsible for hepatitis. But milk thistle seems to reduce inflammation triggered by hepatitis viruses. Inflammation contributes to liver damage and symptoms.

Milk thistle rarely causes side effects at the usual dose of 140–400 mg a day. High doses may cause bloating, nausea, indigestion and diarrhoea.

Liquorice

Many people now think of liquorice as long 'laces', Catherine wheels, 'allsorts' and other sweets. However, our ancestors used liquorice as a medicine even before the rise of the ancient Babylonian and Egyptian civilizations, both of which valued the plant highly.

A chemical called glycyrrhizin in liquorice reduces inflammation, mops up free radicals, modulates the immune system and protects the liver from paracetamol, carbon tetrachloride and other toxins. Furthermore, liquorice seems to attack several parasites, bacteria and viruses, including hepatitis A, B and C, and may help

NAFLD. While further studies are needed, liquorice seems to offer a valuable liver 'tonic'.

Liquorice can cause several adverse events, especially at high doses, including dangerous increases in blood pressure, abnormal changes in heart rhythm, headache, short-lived visual loss, muscle weakness and, ironically, liver damage.

Garlic

A growing number of studies suggest that garlic may help liver diseases. In experiments using rats, S-allylmercaptocysteine (a chemical in garlic) reduced, for example, NAFLD-induced liver injury, fat accumulation and levels of free fatty acids. In rats, raw garlic reduced accumulation of some heavy metals (including cadmium and mercury) in the liver. In experiments, garlic extracts can reverse fibrosis, regenerate liver tissue and restore hepatic function. So, use garlic liberally in your cooking.

11

Living with liver disease

You can reduce the risk that liver disease will progress by, for example, cutting down on alcohol, eating a healthy diet and taking your drugs as recommended by your doctor. This chapter looks at some other ways that may help you live with liver disease.

Quit smoking

In 2014, about one in six adults smoked, increasing their risk of, for example, cancers, strokes and heart disease. Quitting reduces your likelihood of developing most smoking-related diseases. And it's never too late: a 60-year-old gains three years of life by quitting.

Most smokers want to quit. However, only one smoker in 30 quits each year, and more than half relapse within a year. Cutting back seems to increase the likelihood that you'll eventually quit. But people who cut back usually inhale more deeply to get the same amount of nicotine. So, while cutting back helps, don't stop there.

NRT and e-cigarettes

Nicotine's withdrawal symptoms can leave you irritable, restless and anxious, and experiencing insomnia. Withdrawal symptoms are at their worse for two weeks or so. The craving can last longer. Nicotine replacement therapy (NRT) can help you cope. Talk to your pharmacist or GP to find the right combination.

- Patches reduce withdrawal symptoms and craving, but have a relatively slow onset.
- Nicotine chewing gum, lozenges, inhalers and nasal spray act more quickly than patches.

If you still find quitting tough, doctors can prescribe other treatments.

Many people have also quit using e-cigarettes. These don't contain the cancer-causing chemicals laden in tobacco smoke. But as these deliver nicotine, they remain addictive and we still don't know if there are any long-term health risks. So, again, e-cigarettes can take you a large step towards kicking the habit, but you should still aim to quit.

Tips that may make life easier

- Set a quit date.
- Keep a diary of problems and situations that tempt you to light up, such as stress, coffee or pubs. Then find alternatives.
- Try to find something to take your mind off smoking. If you find yourself smoking when you get home in the evening, try a new hobby or exercise. If you find car journeys boring without a cigarette, listen to an audio book or a comedy CD.
- Smoking is expensive. Spend at least some of the money you save on yourself.
- Get a free 'quit smoking' pack from the NHS Smoking Helpline (0800 022 4 332).
- Ask if your area offers NHS anti-smoking clinics, which offer advice, support and, when appropriate, a supply of NRT.

- Think about hypnotherapy: ask your doctor for a recommendation or contact the British Association of Medical Hypnosis (<www.bamh.org.uk/>).

On some measures, nicotine is more addictive than heroin or cocaine. So, regard any relapse as a temporary setback, set another quit date and try again. It's also worth trying to identify why you relapsed. Once you know why you slipped you can try to stop the problem.

The emotional turmoil

Liver disease can be distressing, debilitating and even disabling. If you have cirrhosis, you may live in fear that your liver disease will get worse. Liver cancer may mean that you have to come to terms with your mortality. Not surprisingly, many people with liver disease develop psychiatric problems, such as depression and anxiety. In addition, interferons (page 20) and hepatic encephalopathy (page 8) can trigger depression. Unfortunately, people living with depression or anxiety are often less motivated to stick to their lifestyle regimens and treatments. So, their liver's condition can decline.

If symptoms markedly affect your daily life, your doctor may suggest antidepressants or drugs to alleviate anxiety (anxiolytics). Don't dismiss drugs. It's often difficult to overhaul your lifestyle to help control your liver disease in particular or tackle your life problems while carrying the burden imposed by depression or anxiety.

While drugs can ease depression and anxiety, they do not cure the problem. Rather, putting yourself back in control of your problems is one of the best ways to beat anxiety and depression. On the other hand, feeling that your problems control you is one of the most common causes of anxiety, depression and stress. Talking to a counsellor may help you find new ways to live with chronic liver disease, reduce unhealthy behaviours (such as alcohol abuse), tackle problems more generally and put your affairs in order. They'll help you question the feelings, thoughts and behaviours associated with liver disease that are unhelpful and unrealistic and replace these with approaches that help you actively address your problems and live a more fulfilled life.

Contact the British Association for Counselling and Psychotherapy (<www.bacp.co.uk>) or ask your doctor's surgery if they can recommend a local counsellor. If you are terminally ill try talking to your spiritual leader, a cancer or liver specialist or hospice, or, if you have liver cancer, contact Cancer Research UK (<www.cancerresearchuk.org>) or Macmillan Cancer Support (<www.macmillan.org.uk>).

Tackling stress

Starting to tackle stress now can help bolster your defences when things get tough. There are several ways you can keep your stress levels down:

- As 'first aid', breathe in deeply through your nose for the count of four; hold your breath for a count of seven; breathe out for a count of eight. Repeat a dozen times.
- Yoga, exercise, massage, aromatherapy, reflexology, acupressure, t'ai chi, mindfulness and meditation may alleviate symptoms such as tiredness and sore muscles, aid relaxation, improve mood and reduce anxiety.

- Many herbs can help with fatigue and stress; speak to a medical herbalist.
- Hypnosis can also help with pain, alleviate stress and help you overcome harmful habits such as abusing alcohol, comfort eating or smoking. Some people also find that self-hypnosis helps. Numerous DVDs, CDs and books can help you create the 'focused attention' that underpins hypnosis.
- Learn some relaxation techniques. There are plenty of books, websites, CDs, DVDs and Blu-rays offering suggestions. In addition, many adult education and sports centres offer relaxation courses and lessons. So you should be able to find a technique that works for you.

Tips for a good night's sleep

Everyone with chronic liver disease needs to get a good night's sleep. Fatigue increases the risk of depression in people with HCV. In people with primary biliary cirrhosis, fatigue increases the likelihood of anxiety and depression. The following should help you sleep:

- Wind down or relax at the end of the day: don't go to bed while your mind is still racing or pondering problems.
- Try not to take your troubles to bed with you. Brooding makes problems seem worse, exacerbates stress, keeps you awake and, because you're tired, means you are less able to deal with your difficulties. So, try to avoid heavy discussions before bed.
- Don't worry about anything you've forgotten to do. Get up and jot it down (keep a notepad by the

bed if it's a persistent problem). This should help you forget about the problem until the morning.

- Go to bed at the same time each night and set your alarm for the same time each morning, including the weekends. This helps re-establish a regular sleep pattern.
- Avoid naps during the day.
- Avoid stimulants, such as caffeine and nicotine, for several hours before bed.
- Don't drink too much just before bed as this can mean regular trips to the bathroom.
- An alcoholic nightcap can help you fall asleep. But as blood levels fall, sleep becomes more fragmented and lighter, and you may wake in the latter part of the night. Many people with liver disease shouldn't drink alcohol in any case.
- Don't eat a heavy meal before bedtime.
- Although regular exercise helps you sleep, exercising just before bed can disrupt sleep.
- Use the bed for sex and sleep only. Don't work or watch TV.
- Make the bed and bedroom as comfortable as possible. Invest in a comfortable mattress, with enough bedclothes; make sure the room is not too hot, cold or bright.
- If you can't sleep, get up and watch TV or read, nothing too stimulating, until you feel tired. Lying there worrying about not sleeping keeps you awake.

The ripples from liver disease

Friends, families and wider social networks are essential for most people to enjoy good health and effectively manage serious diseases, including liver conditions. However, the ripples from a serious disease spread throughout the family. Partners shoulder an especially heavy burden. They may fear being alone if the other person dies. They may worry that they could catch the hepatitis virus during sex. They may need to take precautions to prevent the virus spreading. They may face prejudice from neighbours or 'friends'. Sometimes alcohol or drug abuse stretches the relationship to breaking point.

Nevertheless, the practical and emotional support of your family and friends is invaluable if you are trying to quit smoking or drinking, change your diet or cope with the psychological burden. Your partner can help you adopt a healthy lifestyle by changing the shopping list or exercising with you. He or she can ignore bad moods triggered by withdrawal or some treatments for liver disease, boost your motivation and watch for harmful behaviours, anxiety and depression.

Caring for a person with liver disease can be physically demanding and emotionally draining. So, reassure your partner that it's important not to feel guilty about taking time out. Partners of people with liver disease may also feel angry, guilty or resentful. Don't let them bottle these feelings up: they should talk to you, friends, family or a counsellor.

Coming to terms with liver disease is rarely easy. But you don't need to feel that you're chained to a rock, the disease pecking away at your healthy liver. An active, enquiring approach helps loosen the shackles of liver disease. I wish you well.